No-Thing

Every-Thing

Just Living the

Freedom of Unknowing

Also by Jim Galbraith

The Freedom of Unknowing

No-Thing

Every-Thing

Just Living the

Freedom of Unknowing

Jim Galbraith

©2018 by Jim Galbraith

All rights reserved

ISBN—13: 978-0692104637

ISBN—10: 0692104631

for

Wind Through Trees

Contents

Preface

We got off our motorcycles and began a spontaneous climb of Mount Hood in the state of Oregon. It was the late sixties, with blue skies, warm weather and good friends, on one of those perfect days in June.

It wasn't long before I found myself alone on a knife edge of rock and hard snow. On the right was a seventy-degree slope; the left side even steeper. There were the sounds of crunching snow underfoot, the point of my walking stick as it found purchase on the ice, and the wind on my face. The brain was quiet and still.

Mini avalanches of tiny ice crystals tinkled down the steep slopes, a spectrum of color and brilliant reflection, set in motion with a slight flick of the wrist; the sharp end of the walking stick doing the rest.

The body and mind were, peculiarly, absent.

From out of nowhere, it seemed, two words arose—*just living*. There was no brain or body left for any kind of interpretive summation; therefore, it did not seem strange or unusual, that the jingle of ice crystals, and those two words was akin to a realization by nobody.

Then, there was the brain and the body. Then, there was laughter. Then, there was the thought, "This is what life is all about".

Just living.

Laughter and light joy accompanied those two words.

Climbing the mountain stopped.

I made my way to a house sized boulder that was bare on one side, and rich with electric green colors on the other. Gazing into the vastness, deep joy and bliss appeared as the infinite.

Just living!

From far below, my pal Richard, painstakingly, made his way to that rock.

"I don't want to bother you, he said, but I need a light... do you have a match?"

Laughter, comradery, pure air and the uncompromising joy of *just living* lasted for hours, as we sat gazing into apparent infinity.

We made our way back down the mountain, got on our motorcycles and cruised back to Portland.

That was it! On that knife edge was the realization of a lifetime; but where did it go?

It seems that the bulk of my adult life has been spent trying to get that back; attempting to get back *just living*.

I thought that I could search and retrieve the truth of what was there and, ironically, not there.

How cruel to get only a glimpse of the ecstatic, and then having to face the seeming reality of the day to day *grind* early Monday morning.

Today, fifty apparent years later, a book is being written. Who knows what will result?

No one will write, think, gaze, rest, snack, laugh, exercise, edit, format, lose everything or get angry. All the cool stuff, inherent in the seeming writing process, will simply just happen for nobody.

Since no one is writing, a fresh surge of generally nothing, seeming to appear as specifically everything, might emerge; yet, generally everything, apparently arising from precisely nothing, may rush unseen shores of that which is and is not.

There is no 'me' who is present or aware that there is no 'me'; therefore, a book is simply written.

For a brief period of apparent time, all those seeming years ago, there was no 'me', no time and no space. It was heaven on earth.

Now, that apparent divinity, is all that is happening all the time! The only influences now are good food, exercise, plenty of sleep and the wondrous joy and pain of *just living*.

There will be an attempt in this book to speak to you from this unknown place that is not a place. It can be called unknowing, but how can unknowing be called anything?

What seems to work best for the apparent 'me' is unconditional love. All, it seems, that 'I' ever wanted was to be loved, and to know that 'I' was capable of loving.

When the apparent 'Jim' seemingly disappeared, one cloudy day, all that prevailed was love and, paradoxically, all that did not remain was love!

These words are being written, and there appears to be a person writing. Isn't it unusual that you are reading a book written by no one?

'I' still respond to the name 'Jim', still have a social security number, pay taxes and bills, stay updated on the news, grocery shop and change the oil in my car every five thousand miles.

Nothing has really changed, except for one thing:

Everything!

This may seem like a facetious statement, but it's as close to the truth of this communication as 'I' can get.

No-thing has changed; every-thing has changed.

The apparent 'Jim' is no longer, and never was in the first place. A bubbling of nothing, is a book being written, in the perfect disguise of everything.

No-Thing

Every-Thing

Just Living the

Freedom of Unknowing

Introduction

Throughout this book *I, me,* or *self,* as we commonly refer to ourselves and believe as real, is represented as 'I', 'me', 'self', 'Jim', etc. Apostrophes are used to connote the apparent **falseness** of this assumption and, most importantly, to imply that this self is **illusory**; it is not what it seems to be.

That which is literally real, cannot be described in words, and more akin to unfathomable aliveness, wholeness or unconditional love, is represented by the word 'This'. Apostrophes are used to suggest the depth and beauty of 'This' which is already the case.

'I' or 'me' is illusory; it is a creation of the brain. Its complicit partner, the body, supports this illusion with an indefatigable resolve.

'This' euphoric, unconditional love, is all there is and, paradoxically, all there is not; it is an inexplicable, effervescence of aliveness.

There is no story line in this book and so, obviously, it does not have to be read from beginning to end. Each title is an attempt to write of that which is just happening. It, of course, is not possible, because thought and bodily actions merely echo that which is already the case.

The language, herein, appears enigmatic and strange. To say no one wrote this book, and no one will read it, is puzzling; it appears entirely nonsensical.

What is implied has no proof, agreement or direction. The writing is fraught with paradox, due to the limitations of language attempting to describe unencumbered freedom. Words and phrases appear, but it is not possible to make sense out of that which cannot be described.

It is impossible to use dual language in describing that which is non-dual.

'This', which is everything and nothing already, obviously, cannot be described or known.

To illustrate:

When the 'I'/'me' is no more, it is recognized, by no one, that it never was in the first place; or all there *is*, **is** 'This', which is no-thing and every-thing simultaneously.

It may sound comical and could seem condescending to say, "Recognized by no one". The fact is, there is a buoyant recognition, but it is not an experience, feeling or intuition by the seeming 'I' or 'me'.

Inherent in this writing is unknowing and, of course, no one knows this. There is nothing left **to** know there is nothing left.

When the apparent 'Jim' seemingly disappeared 'he' did not know that 'he' had gone, what's more, there was no knowledge that 'he' ever was in the first place! Again, there was nothing left that could know.

Unknowing is, of course, unknowable. The apparent person 'Jim' seemingly disappeared, and the indescribable freedom of that seeming disappearance is unfathomable. Laughter, joy and pain seem to be all that is left; of course, they aren't even left, rather, they seem to arise. Therein, lies the crux of this communication: **the inconceivable joy and pain of just living the freedom of unknowing.**

Every passage is composed with nothing in mind. Words arise and possibly form into phrases or sentences, but may not. There is just writing happening. One could imply, 'This' is freedom writing.

Apparent is used often on the following pages to mean seemingly real or true, but not necessarily so. Seeming and ostensible will also be used for the same purpose.

For example: The apparent 'me' believes it is real. A seeming book is written. Ostensible readers may enjoy perusing a work that implies categorical unknowing.

Happiness and sadness, joy and pain, euphoria and misery are just a few of the words that could be used in the attempt to communicate this perplexing message. The simplicity of unknowing is the joy and woe of aliveness. What is being said, could be described as unconditional love laughing or crying, in pleasure or pain; it is what is, and, of course, what is not.

When there is nothing left, life could seem to be over. What is being put forth, for consideration on the following pages, is just the opposite.

The richness of 'This' aliveness is an indescribable, empty-fullness, resonating concurrently, as no-thing and every-thing.

Are You Kidding Me?

How could it be otherwise?

How could something that does not exist in the first place, suddenly disappear? Impossible.

Of course, I am kidding you. If there is a 'you', and 'you' believe 'you' are real, this book will read and sound like unequivocal nonsense.

This communication might as well be called the bullshit of non-duality; just one sentence of cast iron crap after another.

There is no 'me' and no 'you', but if you believe there is a 'you', that belief will keep you ripe with questions and shrouded in doubt.

How could you believe any of what is being said in this communication? It is

7

unbelievable. What is being said will seem like meaningless, indisputable double-talk.

You would be better off listening to a snake oil salesman, rather than reading one more word of incontrovertible balderdash..

Do you think 'I' care if you get any of what is being said in this discourse? How could 'I', or how could you get this? It must sound like combinations of unintelligible, guttural utterances?

There is nothing to get and nothing to understand.

If you believe you can get 'This', which is everything already. Good for you! I can give you names of those that have taken my money, my time, my love, my sincerity, and have lined their pockets with my apparent longing to finally *"get it"*.

'Jim' is gone, but 'he' was never here in the first place. What kind of a statement is that? How can you get or understand that? Insulting, to say the least, to your high intelligence and complete understanding of this world.

You are being kidded. Anyone who tells you otherwise, is a liar. That which is not real, but pretends to be real to help you get, what can't be gotten, is a charmer.

These words do not arise from something 'Jim' knows. My god! How could 'I' know anything? 'I' do not exist!

'Jim' could not disappear, 'Jim' never was. There was nothing that could vanish; obviously, nothing happened!

Are **you** kidding 'me'?

'I' know you think 'you' are real. No 'I' don't know that. You see? How could 'I' know that? 'I' know nothing. There is no 'I' to know.

Anything is possible in 'This' freedom of unknowing.

Back and forth, up and down 'we' go. 'I' am right, no 'I' am not. How could 'I' be either. There is no 'I' to be 'me'.

Yet, here 'I' am, "Ta-duh"! Writing is happening and 'I' am doing the writing. Well, no 'I' am not. How could 'I'?

Nothing to get my friend. Don't be fooled by anyone. 'This' aliveness is all there is and is not, and it is 'This' already!

Be So Far Away

Years ago, a self-professed, *wise old man*, advised me to stay far away:

Stay far away from family; they mold you into an image of themselves and expect you to act as their mirror for a lifetime.

Stay far away from friends; they expect you to act on their behalf, direct you according to their own needs and wishes, and will use you to make themselves happy.

Remain at great distance from teachers; they, like parents, press you into shallow crevices and expect you to achieve according to their, so-called, standards.

Create vast space between you and all religions, and religious zealots; they will devour your pure and precious heart.

Keep far away from politicians and governments; political agenda's breed sorrow, contempt and false patriotism.

Finally, be so far away you don't even know who or where you are yourself.

This, apparent, *wise old man*, was speaking from, what is commonly referred to as the *higher self*, but nonetheless, the illusory self!

The freedom of unknowing resonates as the obvious: there is no self to be far away!

Sorry *old man*, there is no need to transcend this world.

When the 'I', 'me', 'self' is no more, and recognized that it never was in the first place, high advice is irrelevant. The lower and higher self are creations of the brain and, as such, are illusory.

There is no one to mold, convert, usurp or corrupt.

There is no one left to please parents or satisfy teachers.

There is no one left to seemingly awaken and *know*.

There is no one left to be far away, even from an apparent self.

Everything is 'This' already.

Perfect freedom, not here or now, up or down, near or far.

Undaunted is 'This', which is and is not.

Just living, resonating as no-thing and every-thing simultaneously, is 'This' dis-imprisonment, 'This' glorious aliveness!

Song of Breathing

♫

U uh ∴ *Huh*

U uh ∴ *Huh*

U uh ∴ *Huh*

U uh ∴ *Huh*

The simplest song of unconditional love seeming to rise and fall, *rise and fall,* **rise and fall...**

No 'me' or 'I', just the rhythm of life appearing for no one.

'This' holy breath, this normal breath, this miraculous breath, is all there is and is not.

The guru will tell you to focus on this breath, follow this breath, be one with this breath, meditate on this breath.

An apparent body breathes. This marvel is simply what's happening for no one. It is already no-thing and every-thing. It is already what is and is not.

There is no 'self' *in here* to focus or concentrate on 'This', which is always already the case; yet, most people believe there is such an entity—within.

The breath simply rises and falls, *rises and falls*, **rises and falls,** for no one.

This breath is magnificent wholeness; it is no-thing appearing as every-thing.

The joy of not having to focus on the breath, or any of the other, seeming *ten thousand things,* is a freedom that cannot be expressed in words. The gratitude and the ecstasy cannot be crafted into phrases and sentences.

The breath is the delight of unknowing, the wondrous mystery of *just living.*

Wholeness simply appearing as a living, breathing human being. No in or out, up or down, right or wrong, space or time; just magnificent, unconditional love appearing as breathing.

Such arrogance to think that something illusory could concentrate on that which is and is not.

The apparent breath is always already the case. It is free to appear as breathing, but that is a loose term for the unknown.

Breathing apparently happens for no one:

Its seeming song, an apparent simple crescendo, brief pause at the top, and an unadorned, decrescendo in perfect tune, balance and harmony. It pauses briefly at the seeming bottom, only to begin a fresh, new, satisfying ascension.

Joy of Shaving

"This is just so weird."

- Looking into a mirror
- lathering the face
- hot water on the razor
- starting at the upper lip, moving the double edge blade up and down quickly and accurately
- rinsing the blade
- cruising on to all areas of the face

Laughter and awe arise.

"This feels so good," 'I' say aloud.

Shaving is happening, but there is no 'me' doing a thing!

There is no 'me' standing here knowing there is no 'me' standing here shaving.

Laughter...

...more laughter.

The pleasure of simply shaving is all there is.

There is looking into the eyes of the apparent person named 'Jim', but there is no inside looking out. There is just the wonder and mystery of pure aliveness.

· Rinsing the face with hot water.

"Man, that feels good!"

The image in the mirror appears to smile back and laugh.

The simplicity of *just living* rings as the joy of shaving.

"This is as good as it gets!"

A Room

A white cat sitting on the window sill. A black dog lying on the floor. Sun light, voices, a car passes. New buds of spring, barking dogs. A crow cackles.

Apparent sounds, sights, smells and feelings seem to appear and disappear, rise and fall; an aliveness happening for no one.

The feel of the chair in this room not often used.

The slightest noise triggers dog barking. The thought, "Maybe boredom is a factor, they are animals, but perhaps the human world has altered their instincts," arises.

The beauty of every-thing and no-thing is this naturally, peaceful scenario. Nothing happening; yet, everything is happening.

The thought arises, "Will have to get a chair."

New voices in seeming other rooms.

The glorious nature of *just living* is 'This', an inexplicable aliveness bursting with beauty.

A brief conversation with Max and Jonna. Smiling, laughing, questions and comments regarding non-duality ensue.

'This' is it. 'This' is all there is, all that is happening and, of course, all that is not happening.

No having to add or delete anything.

What could be added to that which is everything and nothing already?

I'll be Happy When...

"I'll be happy when I get that new job and that new motorcycle."

"I'll be happy when I sell this motorcycle, quit this new job, drop out of society and live a content life in the mountains."

"I'll be happy when I get out of this relentless mountain cold, move back to the city and have access to running water."

"I'll be happy when I quit this ridiculous new sales job, move out of this cracker box apartment, and live the *free* life again."

The endless "I'll be happy when" scenario screams at us, prods, probes, and makes tyrannical demands, for many of us, day in and day out. It presents itself in innumerable ways, but its drive is always the same. 'Me', perpetually, looks forward to the next thing; it springs ahead to that which it believes is going to deliver the inevitable prize of peace, contentment and happiness.

All along, that which the apparent 'I' is searching for is 'This' already. That which is longed for is the longing itself, the pain in its apparent experience, the current words being spoken.

There can be no future happiness—ever!

Miraculously, for some apparent people, the 'I' character seems to drop away, and all it has ever longed for, or dreamed of, reveals itself as 'This' already. Happiness, peace, contentment and joy are already 'This', in which the 'me' tenaciously seeks!

The 'I' illusion fades; it is recognized as never having been in existence in the first place!

Peace, happiness and contentment are revealed as the joy of just living.

There is no now or then or will be.

There is simply 'This' which cannot be explained, pointed to or sought.

We, you, us are sincere. We do want, yearn and pray for the truth of this existence.

If we could only know that the yearning, wanting, longing and praying is already 'This' we, apparently, seek. Geographical changes, relationships, mind altering trances, religions, philosophies, ideologies, gurus, self enquiries become instantly irrelevant!

Just living the freedom of unknowing is this unknown knowledge. No need to even get out of bed. Simply enjoy the warmth and comfort of 'This' which is already the case.

Off the Grid

Rustic living in remote areas seems to be popular. Get way out there, away from civilization, and make videos to prove your prowess.

Perhaps, if you are far enough *off the grid,* you will find what you are looking for and be able to tell us about it.

Be a cast away on a desert island, a hermit in the Yukon, raise a family in a rustic log cabin, or simply wander the world as a beggar seeking alms. The result will always be the same--a **story.**

The story of 'me' seeking the freedom of a *blue lagoon,* the happiness of a *hand-built log cabin, enlightenment* in orange robes.

'Me' against insurmountable odds. 'Me' and our happy off the grid home, 'Me' in bliss, 'me', 'me', 'me'...

'Me' will never find what it is looking for. How could it? It is not real.

'Me' refuses to see that 'me' is the problem. It cannot see, know, or experience that it is illusory.

Off the grid it goes looking for that which it will never find.

Just living the freedom of unknowing puts all the unrest, longing, searching, hoping, and dreaming into sweet repose.

The apparent 'Jim', it seems, is so far off grid, free falling so fast, there is absolutely no chance for a 'me' or an 'I'; but saying it like that gives one hope that, maybe, there is a 'me' or an 'I' to be far away or to be in free-fall

There is not.

'This' is unparalleled remoteness at its pinnacle. *Just living* this freedom is the rustic cabin, the blue lagoon, the blissful devotee, the dream come true.

...but, no one knows that. There is no experience, no story to tell, no words to describe 'This' aliveness.

Consequently, there is no showing you how to get here or there or anywhere, because there is nowhere to get to!

A book is being written.

Just living is 'This' which is happening and not happening simultaneously.

'This' is all there is and is not.

'This' is no-thing and every-thing.

How would or could anyone ever find 'This'?

Impossible!

'This' is it already.

No search necessary.

Two Hundred Miles

·Humming tires at seventy-five miles per hour.

·Rushing wind.

·Feel of eyes moving continually in multiple directions.

·Apparent road ahead, to the left, right and rear.

·Driving happening.

·Hands on steering wheel, feet on floor, letting it ride in cruise control.

·Thoughts arise.

·A carrot is eaten.

The question surfaces, "Can an average of sixty miles per hour all the way be sustained?"

•Images of an apparent past seem to appear and disappear.

•Matching the hum of the engine with the voice; then the sound of the tires.

Strangely, no one is driving. There is no awareness. There is just, apparent, driving happening.

There is no 'I' or 'me' taking issue with any of these thoughts.

A large truck appears in the rear-view mirror. The driver is making movements with his hands and head.

Changing lanes and letting him cruise by unfolds quickly.

Most people would say this is being aware, but awareness does not show up.

Instead, what seems to resonate for no one, is simple contentment, as seeming broken white lines whiz by.

No-thing appearing as an extended drive; but no one is driving, and there are no others, seemingly, out there.

What is and is not, as a state trooper aims a radar gun directly at the windshield.

• Instinctive slowing down.

• Chuckling, as the brain issues the thought, "He's already got me."

Every-thing is the same, but everything has changed, arises in the apparent mind.

• Munching on a juicy, organic apple, as a rain squall patters the windshield.

Thumbs, instantly, go to work adjusting the controls for *intermittent* wiper blade action.

No thoughts necessary, but thinking happens.

• Movement, sans presence or awareness.

Driving is fluid and natural.

With no 'me' or 'I' riding along, reaction time is much quicker and more accurate, apparently.

"Change oil when back home," appears in the apparent brain.

Almonds, organic figs and dates are savored, chased down with filtered water.

No music. Just the sound of the tires on the road, hum of the engine, and the wind over the car, accompany no one, averaging sixty-two miles per hour, including a full rest stop, for two hundred miles.

Black Dog

He is always so excited to see me. I leave for a while, but it is, as if, I have never left.

He knows that regular walks, *off leash,* happen when I am around.

I sit in my room, he sits beside me; walk down the hall, he's alongside; I move. He moves.

Right now, I am reading these words to him; he appears to be paying attention.

The pronoun "I" is used; yet, there is no 'I' who sits or walks. Alas, the limitations of dualistic language attempting to describe that which is non-dual.

It could be said that *one walks the dog,* or *no one walks the dog,* or there is just *walking the dog.*

For easier and smoother reading the first-person pronoun "I" or "me" is used as a reference point. We are conditioned to respond to our given name, a tool the brain creates for apparent survival.

In the apparent world it is, as if, the tool has taken itself to be real, is convinced of that seeming truth, and is on a real journey in a real world.

The black dog does not identify as a 'self'. We have had many seeming conversations about this, and he listens carefully; but, to my knowledge, he does not identify as an 'I' or a 'me'.

The sheer joy of running in an open field *off leash*, sniffing grass and chasing geese is palpable. I say, "Good boy," and he comes running back. A dog's life is a good life.

Just double checked and asked him, "Is there a 'you' in there?" His response was a yawn, as he curled up on the rug.

It seems that animals are naturally just living the freedom of unknowing; and they are doing well, exceptionally well.

"That-a-boy," as he runs across the grass glancing at me with what seems a big smile.

He walks over to me and appears ready for the walk home.

"Good boy," as I clip his leash to its body harness.

The sound of a woodpecker high in a microwave tower, a chicken clucks, a jet passes overhead, the sounds of dog steps and human steps as we head home.

How can it get better than this?

Move

.

The apparent body, with the name *Jim* pinned to it, exercises.

The *big three:*

Strength with weight training and pull ups.

Suppleness with stretching.

Stamina with hiking, bicycling, and fast walking.

The body squeezes, rotates, and pushes the muscles; with no 'I' or 'me' setting up unrealistic goals and visions of grandeur, exercise is a daily pleasure.

With no ego to have to please, gratify or reward, competition is non-existent; there are no apparent others in which rivalry can germinate.

As these words are written, sitting up straight, pulling in the stomach, rotating the hips, from one side to the other, is happening.

The neck rocks evenly from side to side, then forward and backward.

Stepping onto the front porch, 'I' hop onto the pull up bar and simply hang for a few seconds, drop down, take a few steps, sit down, and resume typing these words.

Exercise happens, it is naturally 'This' inexplicable aliveness.

The lovely body and brain light up with physical challenges. The skin glistens and the eyes sparkle. Laughter comes easy.

Without a 'me' to please, there is just an apparent handsome man sitting and typing these words.

No brag, just fact.

Laughter.

A three second walk to a set of 1090 dumb bells. Set the weight for light and begin the day with overhead presses and deep squats in four fluid movements.

The sky is clear and the mountains glisten with fresh snow.

The early buds of spring are showing more and more certainty that apparent winter is transitioning out of its seeming dormancy.

Push the muscles and squeeze them simultaneously. One can feel the fresh blood nourishing the body **and** the brain.

Fresh, cool, oxygen expands the lungs and invigorates the blood.

'This' is what is happening.

No-thing.

Every-thing.

One seamless whole.

Exercise for no one, and it feels marvelous!

P~ush~

P~ull~

S~queeze~

Breathe deeply, exhale strongly, let the face grimace with apparent exertion, then smile with relief.

No 'me', just the simplicity and joy of apparent movement.

Stand up. Sit down.

Flex. Release. Flex. Release.

Anywhere, anytime, anyhow…

The joy of aliveness!

S~tretch~ every chance you get.

Watch a cat squeeze and stretch often.

Stand up and stretch.

Sit down and stretch.

Lay down and stretch.

Wherever, whenever…

Stamina—get that heart rate up!

Air in the bike tires…

A hundred psi should do it. Push, pull and squeeze the arms, the back and legs in synchronicity, as the mysterious air works its magic, and a tire is inflated.

No 'me'. Stretching, squeezing and pulling happening for no one, as the tire pump becomes the means for exercising large muscle groups.

The thought arises, "OK. It's bike riding time. An easy one. Go easy."

Push, pull, push, pull…

Uh∴ huh, turns to uh∴∴hah, uh∴∴hah, then uh∴ huh, as the apparent

43

breath matches seeming exertion; hills and open space invite the body to catch the wind.

The mountains, sky and water, breeze across the face, the feel of the legs, the heart beating fast and strong; one harmonious whole in movement sans advancement!

No story.

No fear.

Heart Echo

Aliveness radiates through the apparent wrists, chest, feet and hands.

The rhythm of the pulse--solid, constant, aliveness, resonates strongly as every-thing and no-thing simultaneously.

This apparent heart is ordinary, yet, mysterious, as it seems to magically adjust and readjust without thought or direction.

Unconditional love arises as a beating heart.

The brain is nourished, bathed and replenished with every apparent beat.

Boom, boom, boom...

Boom, boom, boom...

Boom, boom, boom...

'This' is all there is and, miraculously, all there is not.

There is not someone sitting here aware or focusing on this apparent phenomenon. It is simply what is happening.

Breathing and smiling, as the pulse of uncompromising, unconditional aliveness resonates automatically for no one!

There is no 'me' taking credit for, what to some, would seem to be acute awareness. There is no 'me' to say, "My heart", no 'me' *to be aware.*

The apparent combination of breathing and the rhythm of the heart is everything and, oddly, nothing.

The breath, to the illusory 'me', seems to be something that comes out of nowhere, is taken into somewhere, and then flows out again into nowhere. Mere conjecture.

'This' is the inconceivable, mysterious, oneness we call breathing, apparently, happening. No-thing and everything in secming living synchronicity—seamless aliveness for no one.

What appears to be the heart, is the simple, non-dual wonder of unconditional love, nourishing an apparent body perfectly.

This is the wonder of dazzling aliveness, in which no one can take credit, for that which appears to be a miracle. There is no 'my' body, 'my' heart, or 'my' breathing. There is just the apparent heart beating, and the breath rising and falling for no one.

Vibrations through apparent ankles, top of hands, middle of hands, head, chest and feet are this flourishing love.

No parts, just one seamless whole, and the apparent rhythm of the echoing heart and the welcoming breath.

Just living the freedom of unknowing!

But, I Have To...

....go to work, get groceries, take care of the kids, pay the bills. Who is going to do all that important stuff, if there is no 'me'? I mean, it all sounds very good to disappear, to be free, to abide in unconditional love; but there is a life to be lived. It sounds almost like you are free of the responsibilities of day to day living.

Better! There is no 'me' to be free of any duties, tasks or functions; no 'I' to have any importance or responsibilities whatsoever. When there is nothing left, there is no 'who' to play any important roles.

There is no one who stands apart, and realizes he or she is free, and abiding in unconditional love. It's over, absolutely terminated, for the apparent 'me'.

'Me' is addicted to itself. It believes in its own, on-going importance. Without 'me', what would happen? If 'I' am gone my family will suffer. No 'me', no life.

Such arrogance!

When the illusory 'me' seemingly drops away, nothing happens. Nothing happens!

Life goes on as before.

There is getting up in the morning, going to work, shopping, taking care of the kids, staying current with the news, balancing the checkbook; the myriad chores of life continue, ad infinitum.

Life happens with or without the 'me'.

Inherent, in the story of 'Jim', a multitude of solid reasons, justifications, rationalizations, ethical motives, ideas, concepts, rules, duties and responsibilities appeared; all built into what seemed like a real me, surviving in a real world.

When the apparent 'Jim' evaporated, the house payment, power and phone bills came promptly each month in the mail. The price of groceries, house insurance and supplies kept increasing. Filling the gas tank still emptied the wallet. The demands of the kids did not relinquish.

There was no 'Jim' left; yet, all bills got paid, the kids remained warm and safe, the best food was enjoyed, gas for the car was purchased with a smile, and all bills were paid *before* they were due.

No-thing was left.

Every-thing was left.

Nothing happened.

No-thing changed.

Every-thing changed.

There was, simply, no 'I', 'me' or 'Jim' making up, living in, or suffering within a story.

When the story ends, no past or future can be found; yet, memories or planning may arise in thought for no one.

Wonderfully, there is no, nor was there ever, 'Jim', to perceive what is or is not.

Heat

Images, words, sounds and harmonies, called thoughts, apparently appear and disappear, surface and vanish, rise and fall, materialize and dematerialize.

The human brain seems to glow--on fire with apparent unlimited capabilities.

Thoughts flash, sparkle and burn. The mind, with the seeming power of the sun, works its magic. It blazes. The breath chills, the heart glows, in an unfathomable dance of stunning aliveness, emanating from nothing.

The brain, perhaps out of necessity created the 'I', the 'me'. Why is it that most of the apparent population of this earth, believe this creation of brain sensors and bodily sensations to be real? Astounding illusory agreement!

The brain does not recognize when the 'I' or 'me' drops away; consequently, when that non-happening occurs the brain does not miss 'me'. There is absolutely no longing or wishing for that *made-up* self to ever return!

It is, as if, the 'I' or 'me' is a veritable anachronism. Perhaps it was once useful to the brain for survival in stark, apparent ancient settings. When it is no more, it is not missed.

Thoughts seem to burn, sparkle and fire with renewed life and vigor. There is no 'me' present and aware to interfere with such fervent heat!

What freedom! My God! What freedom!

There is no 'me' to know 'This', no 'I' to be aware of 'This', no self to be present **or** aware of 'This'.

No-thing, flowering as unencumbered aliveness, seeming to appear as every-thing joyous and free!

This body-mind configuration wants to leap up and fly, screaming out the message:

"This is it already"!

Just living the freedom of unknowing is 'This', which is everything and nothing, crackling clean and smooth, no breaks or gaps, and on fire with well-being and contentment!

Beauty

Nowhere to go. Nothing to do. Alone at the kitchen table. The familiar chairs, colors and sounds of an apparent Thursday afternoon.

Thoughts arising, the feel of the wrists on this keyboard. Stretching the neck, rolling the shoulders, gazing at trees and sky.

Love pouring, from every conceivable angle, the simple joy of being alive.

One does not have to find 'This', seek 'This', yearn or long for 'This', which blooms, in perpetual splendor, for no rhyme or reason.

'This' festive, effervescent, uncorked aliveness, apparently happening for no one, shines.

The perfection is indescribable; yet, once again, writing happens, smiling continues, and the well-being of simple, care-free living seems to unfold.

It is not possible to explain, discuss, or illustrate what is being hinted in these words.

Reds, browns, greens, blacks and grays seem to blend together and appear as an inside room. A window opens to, what seems to be, a forest transitioning out of winter dormancy.

'This', which **is** already, is the mystery. How can one find 'This' which is every-thing and no-thing concurrently?

The beauty of the wind and sky, the body and mind, life and death—all one, only one, just one.

Wholeness, seemingly, appearing and disappearing, rising and falling, laughing and crying or living and dying, is never two.

Just living is and is not 'This' aliveness appearing for no one.

Disturbing Noises

Cartoons playing in the other room. Constant high-pitched voices, boing, boings, heavy drama, screaming, growls, and strange music. It seems to be running, but nobody seems to be watching. It's more of a background for the mind.

It is difficult to think with this harsh, discordant, mixture of sounds.

That same cartoon scenario seems to be the current condition of the apparent world. Humankind apparently lost in a cacophony of real news, fake news, cartoon news which appears as the background, or foreground for billions of people.

The apparent world seems restless, ill at ease—fearful.

All the distractions ever created, lined up and compared, would still all remain simply diversions for the restless mind.

No 'me', no distractions.

No 'I', no fear.

No 'self', This freedom'.

There is no way to tell others of 'This' miraculous, indescribable no-thing, which is 'This' wondrous every-thing.

What is blatantly obvious for no one, is incomprehensible to anyone who believes this self to be real.

It seems that to hear this message, it must be spoken or written; but that is not true. This message cannot be spoken or written!

That which apparently looks, in seeming silence, tries to find the words to describe this obvious aliveness.

It is a sincere effort.

There is no one looking and no one to hear. Isn't it curious that writing of 'This', which cannot be known or understood, is even occurring?

This is the book 'I' want full access to; it looks like 'I' will have to write it. 'I' am not writing it, but a book is being written.

Will 'I' still have that access?

Dark Path

"Better wear those shoes, and tomorrow you will want those for the drive."

"Put those shoes on over there."

Porch light on.

Bags in hand.

The sound of strong wind blasts through the trees. Stars and clouds. Traffic in the distance.

Darkness.

The pace is quick, but the ground is rutted and unstable. Some light here and there.

Across the grass, onto the bark, across the street.

A car with its door and hood open; a man standing in the shadows.

First the recycle bag, then the trash bag into its intended destination.

Back the same way.   A quick turn towards the unexpected red car.

Wind on the face, the rush of its power crashing through the trees.

A familiar porch light.

"Wow!"

Into an *on the grid* shelter, yet an absolutely *off the grid* life.

One might think this is an awareness of a simple walk to empty the trash; however, it is only that which is happening.

There is no awareness, no being in the moment, no meditative contemplation; just the simple beauty of an apparent short walk across the lawn on a dark and windy night.

Unknowing at its best!

Just Loving

Are you loved and capable of loving?

The inherent difficulty, in answering this question, seems to arise with the pronouns "you", "I" and "me".

It's wonderful to be 'me', however, when the illusory 'I' or 'me' tries to love or be loved, difficulties often arise.

We are human. We identify as 'I' or 'me'. If only someone, out of sincere love, could point out the obvious and simple fact: It is not the 'I' that loves, but rather, love itself, loving (always already) every- thing and no-thing simultaneously, unconditionally and without compromise.

There is no separate 'I' loving a separate 'you'. It's perfectly fine to say I love you. It's also fine to hear I love you too.

What is not fine is to believe 'I' am a real 'I' loving an actual 'you'.

The human brain creates the illusory 'me', and then wonders why love seems illusive.

The greatest thing we can do as human beings is to recognize the illusory nature of the 'I' or 'me', and simply let love, be love, as love, *unconditionally*.

This is the recognition we had as babies; but conditioning, by well-meaning others, seemed to divide this sweet, indivisible whole in half. Once divided, the two became four, and the four became eight...

The pain of this apparent separation is relevant. We, as adults, must inform our children of the illusory nature of this seeming separation.

Unfortunately, most people seem to separate into the illusory self, and stay in that appearance for an entire life time!

It is, therefore, impossible for most adults to simply let love reveal itself to the child in two ways that are not ways:

•The non-discovery, that he or she is loved unconditionally, and he or she is that love already.

•He or she is capable of sharing love without any stipulations, conditions or barriers, for love is all there is and is not.

It is fine to identify as 'I' or 'me', for that is what we do as human beings. We use pronouns to communicate.

What is not fine, is to believe and agree with countless others, that this 'I' or 'me' is real, and that it can do something about the predicaments it currently finds itself in.

We all need help in knowing we are loved when we are immersed in the illusory, separate state of the 'I' or 'me'.

With the demise of the illusory 'I', 'me' or 'you', nothing is rediscovered; there is just 'This', unconditional love, which is always already the case.

'That', which is 'This', always already, is recognized, by no one, to have never been separate in the first place!

It is so easy and obvious, but for most people, this communication falls on deaf ears.

Love is all that 'This' is, and all that 'This' is not.

The mystery of 'This', which is and is not, is, of course, incomprehensible.

Just living is just loving.

Love is just living the freedom of unknowing.

Sincere

'I' just don't have anything to say. The only word arising is sincere. Am 'I' sincere, are 'you' sincere, is 'anyone' sincere?

Just living the freedom of unknowing does not answer the question of sincerity; but what appears to surface is the essence of sincerity, which is love.

The ultimate gift, of course, is love. To help someone know they are loved, and capable of love themselves is inherent in *just living*.

Guidance counseling need not be given, nor direction or advice, for love is always already. Simply living as love, in love, for love and only love **is** what is, and is not.

Love cannot be described, known or experienced; yet, it is sincerity itself, reality itself, unfeigned honesty itself. That which is and is not already!

So, ultimately, it is not possible to show someone he or she is loved, since there is no one to do the showing, and no one to be the one shown.

Love is and is not. It is a mystery.

What is apparently being attempted, in voicing these incomprehensible statements, is sincerity itself. There are no positions being taken, and no guidance being given; yet, love is the essence of what is, and is not, being suggested.

When the 'I' is recognized to be illusory, all that apparently remains is every-thing and no-thing; the only word that seems to work in this dichotomy is love.

The average person seeks, longs for, desires, dies for this love, which seems illusive and unobtainable; yet, it is already 'This' which is sought or wished.

No one can show us we are loved, nor can they show us we are capable of love.

Love shows us we are loved.

Love shows us how to love.

Love shows us we are capable of love.

That's not quite right either, for there is no 'we' or 'us'. There is simply, love.

'We' can call it love. 'We' can call it happiness. 'We' can call it anything 'we' like, but that would not be it.

The marvelous joy, of just living the freedom of unknowing, is the mystery of living in the sincerity of pure aliveness!

Peace and Quiet

If there was a way to show, just one person, the immensity of peace, and the depths of quiet, inherent in this aliveness, it would be done.

How could wholeness do that? It would have to separate into one, and then another, to do so.

'This' **is** peace and quiet. It cannot be shown. It already is 'This'.

Apparent sounds and reverberations arise the moment we wake up in the morning. Noise bombards our senses in a relentless barrage of natural and unnatural cacophony.

The blare of a siren is undeniably shrill, the drone of a leaf blower, skull numbing, a dog barking from sun up to sun down, frays the nerves.

The seeming racket of an apparent world appears to stagger the strongest people.

When the 'I' is no more, uncomfortable noise fallout has nothing to stick to, and seems to, simply, be just what is happening.

Likewise, the indescribable peace and quiet of billowing aliveness, surges, swells, and rolls in unseen oceans of unconditional love.

Strength and weakness are irrelevant. There is, simply, walking straight, talking straight, and remaining *in tune* with and as this formless love.

Alas, this miracle, this mystery cannot be shown. It already is what is being looked for. One seeks this, which is already 'This'.

Bombs may fall, bullets might fly, but unconditional love cannot and will not ever be absent. How could that which is, and is not, ever be unavailable?

The tinnitus in 'my' apparent ears is thunderous twenty-four hours a day; yet, the quiet of nothing and everything, roars with the stillness of silence and the hush of peace.

How wonderful to be free of the apparent separation between seeming personalities and ego's. There is just this pristine aliveness, teaming with pleasure and pain, joy and sorrow, happiness and sadness, mysteriously arising for no one.

Nothing Left

When the 'I' collapsed there was nothing left, except for one thing:

Everything.

How, unequivocally, amazing!

First, the apparent, sudden demise of the character known as 'me'.

Then, the recognition, by no one, that there never was an 'I' or 'me' **to** collapse.

Followed by complete unknowing of that which was being suggested.

Topped off with a somewhat peculiar, non-understood recognition, that nothing had changed.

Moreover, no-thing and every-thing were one and the same. There were not two.

Thoughts, feelings and emotions arise. Life has not changed; yet, living has undergone a complete transmutation.

There is no one writing these apparent words. No one sitting on this seeming chair. No one telling these hands what to do.

In the life of 'Jim' there seemed to be awareness of every big or little thing, and with that apparent awareness came interpretations and judgements.

In, 'This' freedom of unknowing, the indescribable quiet of just living is all there is and is not.

Judgements and interpretations may arise, but neither have a place to land and secure themselves. They quickly dissipate, dissolve or evaporate, since there is no host for them to cling to.

So, every-thing is left, yet, strangely, no-thing is left; apparently, being and not being, was and was not in the first place!

To be is and is not to be.

Life appears to happen. Living seems to happen.

Noth↔every↔thing could be a word for no-thing and every-thing:

Noth↔every↔thing is that which is not, and that which is, simultaneously!

The sublime excellence of glorious, mysterious, unconditional, loving aliveness resonates with the simplicity of a quiet Monday afternoon.

Miss Me?

The brain creates the 'me'. It maintains this illusion with a dynamic influence, unparalleled in nature.

When the apparent 'me', the person who identified as 'Jim', was no more; it was, as if, the 'me' or 'I' had no prior existence in the first place!

In terms of time, it has been awhile since the apparent collapse of 'me' took place.

Oddly, 'I', 'Jim', 'me' is not missed, not by someone else; but the brain, responsible for typing these words, creating 'Jim' himself, does not miss 'Jim'!

The brain does not miss 'Jim'!

'My' brain does not miss 'me'.

'I' do not miss 'me'.

There is no 'I', 'me' 'self' or 'Jim' to be missed.

Amazing!

Most people want to know their presence on this earth has been meaningful; and when they are gone, maybe they will be remembered.

That is fine.

When the very brain, that seemed to be the real 'you', does not miss 'you'; how could it **ever** miss someone else?

That does not mean that when a loved one dies, or is injured, there is no pain. Unconditional love may arise as heartbreak and sadness, the likes of which, one has never seen or felt before.

There is simply no 'I', 'me', or self to be missed.

Likewise, there is no 'self', 'I' or 'me' to be missing itself!

The brain has no need to construct, or re-create, another illusion to replace the one it apparently lost.

It is recognized, by no one, that the 'me' can be compared to an outdated piece of software.

How often do we miss our old, antiquated cell phones?

Once gone.

Not missed.

Never was.

No-thing left

Every-thing right.

Oh, 'This' Is Good!

Hot green tea, as the rain falls, refrigerator hums, and the screaming and laughing of children playing, seemingly fills the air.

The greens of organic avocado, kale, fresh parsley, celery, rainbow chard and broccoli--maroon of red cabbage--white of cauliflower--yellow-orange of steaming hot sweet potato and the crimson of tomato, frame 'my' dinner.

Chopped parsley, sage, rosemary and thyme, along with turmeric and cayenne pepper, are added to this delightful sight.

A fresh piece of baked, red, Sockeye salmon, accented with garlic salad dressing, is ready.

So simple to make.

A joy to consume.

The glorious beauty of apples, oranges, bananas and tomatoes grace 'my' kitchen counter top.

'I' open the refrigerator to the myriad colors of fruits and vegetables from around the world.

How can a person be any richer than 'he' or 'she' who has food on the table?

Breakfast earlier this morning arises in thought. Simple muesli and a little protein powder doctored up with: acai, cinnamon, pomegranate and goji powder, vitamin c crystals, chia, flaxseeds, hemp hearts, raspberries, blueberries, chopped banana and a generous pouring of oat milk.

The rain continues to fall on a quiet spring day. A car passes by, there is ringing in the ears; in the distance moving mist caresses the trees.

Noth↔every↔thing happening.

Oh, 'This' is good!

About the Author

Jim Galbraith, a native of the Pacific Northwest, was born in Washington State, and educated at Lewis and Clark College in Portland, Oregon.

When he was seventy, while sitting at his dining room table, life, as he knew it, folded and vanished!

Strangely, as he walked through the kitchen, moments later, there was no sense of a separate inside self perceiving a separate outside world. Inner and outer seemed to be one organic whole.

Stoic, non-experiential, seriousness ensued; something unknown yet familiar, seemed to resonate as unconditional and timeless well being.

It was, as if, death was occurring, or perhaps, this was its aftermath; yet, breathing and smiling was happening!

All that seemed to be known had disappeared.

The brain was lucid, the body intact, but 'Jim' was gone. There was nothing left; yet, everything remained!

Aliveness was all there was, and peculiarly, all there was not.

'Jim' has not reappeared.

No-Thing

Every-Thing is 'his' second book.

No-Thing Every-Thing

P.O. Box 2696

Poulsbo, WA 98370-9998

Printed in Great Britain
by Amazon

53363548R00067